Ketogenic Di

GW01091374

42 Delicious Ketogenic D Loss.

Sara Banks

Table Of Contents

Introduction

I want to thank you and congratulate you for purchasing the book "Ketogenic Diet Recipes-42 Delicious Ketogenic Diet Recipes For Weight Loss"

This book contains proven weight loss ideas and Ketogenic Diet recipes that will help you meet your health and weight loss goals. The Ketogenic diet is one of the most popular diets in the world of weight loss right now for many reasons. Thousands have enjoyed the many health benefits including lower blood pressure, lower cholesterol, more energy, clearer thinking, and of course weight loss. Many also believe and follow the ketogenic diet to fight cancer as well.

Use these recipes and information to help your life turn around towards a healthier and fit you!

Thanks again for purchasing this recipe book, I hope you enjoy it!

Sara Banks

The Ketogenic Diet: An Introduction

If you are struggling with epilepsy, you might have come across a few suggestions referring you to try the ketogenic diet. The ketogenic diet is mainly a low carb diet, with an adequate amount of proteins and very high fats. As such, you can use this diet when you want to lose weight. This diet has a tendency to force your body to burn fats, which are turned into fatty acids and ketone bodies.

Ketogenic diets are mainly based on ketosis, a state in which the body uses ketones from fats for energy, instead of glucose from carbohydrates for several organ functions. Some organs in your body prefer using these ketones instead of glucose for fuel when they are available, like the heart. However, it is important to note that not all ketone molecules can be converted and used as energy, like the acetone, which is excreted from your body through your breath and urine as waste.

You can detect the presence of the acetone molecule from your urine using a dipstick known as ketostix. The stick turns purpler with the increase in acetone levels.

It is sometimes assumed that if your body burns too much fat for energy, then it will not have enough glucose because of the low carbohydrate content in the ketogenic diets. This has however not been proven from the numerous studies done on people on low carb diets. On the other hand, it is important to note that even though your body converts glucose to fat, the reverse is not true. However, your body has the ability to convert some of the proteins you take into glucose instead, and as such is convenient especially for people who are not lactose tolerant.

One of the merits of ketogenic diet is that it prevents you from feeling hungry, which is one of the main reasons people fail to sustain strict diets. In addition, the ketogenic diet has a very low amount of carbohydrates, which results to more weight lose. This is because low carb diets help eliminate excess water from your body, and lower insulin levels, which increases the speed with which kidneys shed excess sodium.

Interestingly though, not all fats are equal. There are some fats stored in the abdominal cavity known as visceral fat that have the tendency to lodge around the abdominal organs. Low carb diets help to reduce these fats, which can cause inflammation, and increase insulin resistance as well as metabolic dysfunction in your body, all of which are rapidly becoming common in Western countries.

Aside from helping to reduce weight, these diets help to lower triglycerides levels, which are caused by excessive consumption of carbohydrates, and are known risk factors for heart disease.

Breakfast Recipes
1. Scrambled Eggs

Ingredients

1 Tablespoon of unsalted butter

3 large eggs

A pinch of salt and freshly ground pepper

Directions

Beat the eggs using a fork.

Using a medium skillet, melt the butter over low heat.

Add the egg mixture.

Gently push the eggs to the center of the pan and allow the watery parts to run out under the region with a flexible spatula. Let them cook while moving the eggs with the spatula until the eggs are set. This can take about 1 1/2 to 3 minutes.

Season with salt and pepper; and serve hot.

2. Ketonnaise

Ingredients

2 egg yolks

1 tablespoon of lemon juice

½ cup of olive oil

¼ teaspoon of salt

1 tablespoon of wine vinegar

1 teaspoon of dry mustard

½ cup of liquid coconut oil or ½ cup of olive oil

1 dash of Tabasco sauce

Instructions

Put everything except the oil in a clean jar and cover.

Combine the two oils in a glass-measuring cup. Keep this ready.

Using a stick blender, blend the egg-yolk mixture for several seconds until it is uniform.

Pour the oil in the blender while still running. Be sure that the stream has the diameter close to that of a pencil lead. Make sure you mix the oil thoroughly in the blender before you stop.

You will know when you are done when the mayo is hard, and there is a puddle of oil on top. It might take all the oil although there may be a little left in the cup. You can use it to fry something later.

3. Asian Noodles

Ingredients

1 packet of traditional shirataki noodles

1 tablespoon of natural peanut butter

1 tablespoon of coconut oil

½ teaspoon of dark sesame oil

1 tablespoon of chicken broth

1 drop of liquid stevia extract or liquid sucralose

½ teaspoon of grated ginger root

1 teaspoon of soy sauce

1 clove of garlic

1 scallion

Instructions

Spill the shirataki noodles into a sink strainer, rinse, and then drain properly.

Put in a bowl and then nuke for about two minutes.

Re-drain and then nuke for an extra minute or two; be sure to drain one more time.

Separate the noodles using kitchen shears. When this has been achieved, put everything but the scallion into the bowl then stir until everything mixes and forms a sauce.

Garnish with the scallion then serve.

4. Lime Cheesecake

Ingredients

8 ounces of softened cream cheese

1 tablespoon of vanilla

½ cup of heavy whipping cream

6 packets of True Lime

3 whole eggs

Artificial sweetener that is equal to 12 teaspoons of sugar

Instructions

Beat the heavy cream and cream cheese using an electric mixer until it forms a smooth mixture. Add the remaining ingredients and blend well.

Pour the batter into ramekin, lined and greased, and put on a cookie sheet. Insert a knife at the center of the mixture then let it bake for 30 to 40 minutes at 350 degrees F until the knife comes out clean.

Place on a rack until it cools and then refrigerate.

You can serve once cooled.

5. Broccoli Cheese Soup

Ingredients

2 cups of broccoli florets

2 cups of water

4 ounces of softened cream cheese

½ cup of chicken broth

¼ cup of heavy whipping cream

1 teaspoon of salt

Pepper to taste

1 cup of Cheddar cheese

Instructions

Steam the broccoli florets until tender. Put all the cream cheese, ½ cup of the broccoli, all the heavy cream and ½ cup of the water in a blender. Mix until it forms a smooth mixture.

Pour this mixture into a large saucepan, and then add the rest of the broccoli, chicken broth, and water. Mix until all the ingredients blend in together. Bring to a simmer over medium heat.

Add the Cheddar cheese when the saucepan has heated and then mix until it melts and consolidates into the mixture. Add pepper to taste.

6. Fat Scramble

Ingredients

1 tablespoon of olive oil

1 egg

2 teaspoons of heavy cream

2 teaspoons butter, melted

1 tablespoon of small ham cubes

Salt and pepper to taste

⅛ cup of Cheddar cheese

Instructions

Beat the egg, cream, salt, pepper and butter together.

Spray a skillet with olive oil and then heat it over medium heat.

Pour the egg mixture into a saucepan and mix until the eggs are almost set using a turner or spatula.

Add cheese and ham while mixing until all the cheese has melted and the eggs are set.

7. Hot Cereal

Ingredients

1½ tablespoons of ground pecans

1 tablespoon of flax seed meal

1½ tablespoons of shredded coconut meat

⅓ cup of boiling water

A pinch of salt to taste

Splenda or your preferred sweetener to taste

2 tablespoons of heavy cream

A dash of cinnamon (optional)

Instructions

Put the flax seed meal, coconut, and pecans in a bowl, and then add salt. Mix by stirring until all the ingredients have blended.

Add boiling water, and stir until it incorporates into the mixture. Leave it for a minute or two and then add the sweetener and cream.

8. Paleo Pudding

Ingredients

3 tablespoons of chia seeds

1 scoop of chocolate protein powder

1 cup of unsweetened almond milk

1 tablespoon of honey (optional)

¼ cup of fresh or frozen raspberries

Instructions

Mix the chocolate protein powder and almond milk, and then stir well using a fork. Add the chia seeds into the mixture then let this blend into the mixture by stirring with a fork. Leave it to rest for about five minutes and then stir.

Let the mixture stay for another five minutes and then stir again before putting in the refrigerator for about thirty minutes to rest.

Serve when it has cooled and add the raspberries at the top.

You can put the left overs in storage containers and refrigerate.

9. Spinach Omelet

Ingredients

4-5 egg whites

2 tablespoons of almond milk, soy milk, coconut milk or skim milk

1 egg yolk

1 handful of shredded spinach

1 plum tomato

a pinch of basil

1 tablespoon of purple onion

Cooking spray

Garlic (optional)

Instructions

Chop the vegetables.

Beat the almond milk, egg whites, and the yolk together.

Spray some oil on a small frying pan and then quickly sauté the veggies until soft.

Set the vegetables aside, spray the pan again, and pour the eggs over medium-low heat.

Cook until the eggs are stiff, add the veggies on one side, fold the eggs on one side and pour the veggies over the top.

Add fruits then serve.

10. Bacon and eggs

Ingredients

1 tablespoon of butter

1 strip peeled carrot

8 slices of meaty bacon

½ cup of finely chopped celery

½ cup of chopped broccoli or cauliflower

½ large white chopped onion

½ cup shredded Colby jack cheese

4 large organic eggs

Instructions

Slice the bacon along the grain to get small strips.

Place the butter in a large skillet over medium heat until it melts then add the bacon and vegetables.

Sauté the vegetables and bacon in the melted butter for about 20 minutes while stirring occasionally until crisps of the bacon form on the edges and the vegetables become tender.

Let the mixture spread over the skillet uniformly, and then divide into quarter sections with trenches between two sections.

Break one egg into each trench and let them cook until the eggs are almost set. If you prefer cooked yolks, you can just cover the skillet to allow the eggs to cook thoroughly.

Just before the eggs are set, daub the cheese at the top and let it cook a little more until all the cheese has melted. Serve while hot.

11. Onion and Cheese Quiche

Ingredients

5-6 cups of shredded muenster

Half Colby jack cheese

1 large finely chopped white onion

2 tablespoons of butter and a little more for greasing the pans

2 cups of heavy cream

12 large organic eggs

1 tsp of ground black pepper

1 tsp of salt

2 tsp of dried thyme

Instructions

Preheat your oven to 350 degrees.

Add butter in a pan over medium heat and melt then add the vegetables and sauté until the onions turn soft and remove from heat, and cool.

Grease two medium size quiche pans. Press 2 cups of the shredded cheese at the bottom of each pan. Add a half of cooled vegetable mixture to each of the pans over the cheese evenly.

Beat 12 eggs into a large mixing bowl. Add the spices, and cream and mix with a whisk until they turn frothy. Pour ½ of this egg mixture over each of the pans, and then distribute the vegetables and cheese over the egg mixture.

Put all the pans into the oven and let them bake for about 20 minutes until they are set.

Serve while hot, or refrigerate or freeze for preservation.

Main Dishes
12. Avocado Turkey Bacon Salad

Ingredients

For the dressing

1 tablespoon of olive oil

1 teaspoon of lemon juice

1 tablespoon organic apple cider vinegar

A little garlic (optional)

1 teaspoon of Dijon Mustard

Salt and pepper to taste

For the Salad

Extra virgin olive oil cooking spray

4 cherry tomatoes

100 grams of ham

2 hard-boiled eggs

30 grams of blue cheese

½ diced avocado

2 cups of coarsely chopped romaine lettuce

2 slices of turkey bacon

Instructions

For the Salad

Hard boil the eggs using the regular method, or a steamer.

Cut the ham into small cubes and then put them in an olive oil sprayed skillet for 3-5 minutes to heat.

Slice the eggs once boiled.

Place lettuce in an empty bowl then add in avocadoes, halved cherry tomatoes, turkey bacon, blue cheese, eggs, and ham, along each other in rows.

Spread the dressing evenly at the top.

13. Beef Scramble And Egg Whites

Ingredients

1 lb extra lean ground beef

2 cups of regular or baby spinach

8 egg whites

½ cup of red peppers

4 small tomatoes

2 Italian tomatoes

Salt & black pepper to taste

Instructions

Preheat an olive oil sprayed pan over medium heat then put the beef in the hot pan and let it break into large pieces.

Divide the beef into smaller pieces while cooking and then put it in a bowl when it has cooked and turned golden brown. Set it aside.

Beat the egg whites and pour them over the cooked meat.

Sauté the spinach, tomatoes, red basil and peppers lightly then place them on top of the meat and serve while hot.

14. Chicken salad

Ingredients

2 cups of baby spinach

½ or 1/3 large Avocado

½ chicken breast

1 tablespoon of Peri Peri Sauce

1 piece of low sodium bacon

Instructions

Heat the pan over medium heat and cook the bacon until it has turned brown and crispy.

Cut the chicken breast into equal parts while cooking. Put the chicken breast slices in the bacon fat and let them cook for 1 minute on one side then turn on the other side and fry for about five minutes. Before the five minutes are over, slice the avocado, and bacon into small pieces.

Put the avocado and spinach in a large bowl, and then add the peri peri sauce and bacon.

15. Ginger Beef

Ingredients

2 sirloin steaks cut in strips

1 small diced onion

1 tablespoon of olive oil

2 small diced tomatoes

1 crushed clove garlic

4 tablespoons of apple cider vinegar

1 teaspoon of ground ginger

Salt and pepper

Directions

Place oil in a large skillet. Once hot, put the steaks and brown them.

Add the garlic, onion, and tomatoes when both sides have been properly cooked.

Mix the ginger salt, pepper and vinegar in a bowl then and add the mixture to the skillet.

Cover the skillet, and maintain low heat. Let this simmer until all the liquids evaporate.

16. Chicken Curry

Ingredients

3lbs of chicken thighs

1 cup of water

7 oz of paneer packet

1/2 cup of heavy cream

1 cup of crushed tomatoes

1 tablespoon of olive oil

4 tablespoons of butter

1 1/2 teaspoon garlic paste

2 teaspoon coconut oil

1 teaspoon coriander powder

1 1/2 teaspoon of ginger paste

1 teaspoon salt

1 teaspoon of garam masala

1/2 teaspoon of paprika

1 teaspoon freshly ground black pepper

1/2 teaspoon of red chili powder

1/2 teaspoon of kashmiri mirch

5 sprigs cilantro

Instructions

Preheat the oven to 375 degrees F.

Rub the chicken thighs with olive oil, salt and pepper to taste then place them on a cookie sheet to roast for about 25 minutes.

Slice the paneer into tiny bits and set aside.

Preheat the pan under medium heat and add the coconut oil and butter. Wait until the butter turns brown and then add garlic paste and ginger. Sauté for about 2 minutes before adding the tomato.

Mix the garam masala, coriander powder, paprika, salt and red chili powder, blend them and simmer until the oil shows on top. Blend in the paneer slowly then add water and let it simmer for 5 minutes.

Stir the mixture under medium low heat and let it simmer until it comes to a boil again.

When the chicken is ready, remove from heat and let the bone apart then dip it in the sauce and mix well. Allow to simmer for another 5 minutes then cilantro to garnish and serve hot.

17. Low Carb Pizza

Ingredients

2 slices of low-carb bread

Cheese, 2 ounces per pita

3 tablespoons of tomato sauce

1 dash of garlic powder (optional)

1 dash of ground black pepper

1 dash of chili flakes (optional)

Optional

2 slices bacon

1 tablespoon of roasted red peppers

1 handful of spinach

½ cup of artichokes/olives/pesto

½ cup of pineapple/ avocado/mango/ Rooster Sauce

1 cup of pepperoni/prosciutto/salami/roast beef/ham

Instructions

Preheat the oven to 450 degrees F.

Spray the bread with cooking spray then put in the preheated oven for about two minutes until it hardens and then toast the crust.

Mix the tomato sauce with the garlic powder, black pepper and chili flakes. When the bread is ready, remove from oven and add the sauce, and then the cheese.

Spread with olive oil and then toast for another 2 minutes at a temperature of 450 degree F until it crisps.

Let it cook for another three-six minutes until the cheese melts completely.

18. Creamed Spinach

Ingredients

10 ounces frozen chopped spinach

2 tablespoons cream cheese

3 tablespoons butter

Salt and pepper

Instructions

Remove the spinach from the freezer and put them in a microwaveable bowl then add 4 tablespoons of water, and then cover. Let these nuke for 8 minutes; check if they are done after the eight minutes- they are bound to be a little cold at the middle, so stir it up and set another 4 minutes on the microwave.

When done, pour in a sink strainer and drain it hard with a spoon. Transfer the spinach to a bowl then add the cream cheese and butter and stir until both melt and are fully consolidated and form a smooth sauce. Add salt and pepper to taste, and then divide into two plates.

19. Meatloaf

Ingredients

½ cup of almond flour

2 cups of shredded and minced cheddar cheese

½ cup of shredded parmesan cheese

2 tablespoons of butter

8 ounces of softened cream cheese

5 minced garlic cloves

8 ounces of chopped white onion

2 large eggs

1 cup of chopped green pepper

1 tablespoon of thyme leaves

1 tablespoon of chopped fresh basil leaves

1 teaspoon of salt

¼ cup of minced parsley leaves

2 teaspoons of Dijon mustard

½ teaspoon of ground black pepper

¼ cup of heavy cream

2 tablespoons of barbecue sauce

2 lbs of ground beef

½ teaspoon of unflavored gelatin

1 lb of Italian sausage

Instructions

Preheat the oven to 350 degrees.

Oil a medium sized baking dish with butter and put aside. Whisk the Parmesan cheese and almond flour in a small bowl and place aside.

Mix the cheddar cheese and softened cream cheese together in another bowl until a butter texture is formed. Place the butter in a medium skillet and melt it over medium heat then add in garlic, onion, and pepper. Let this cook for about eight minutes until they soften. Set aside to cool and start preparing the remaining ingredients. Place the mixture in a food processor when it has cooled enough for a few seconds until the vegetables are minced.

Take another small deep bowl, and blend in the eggs with salt, pepper, spices, BBQ sauce, mustard, and cream. Add gelatin on top and leave it for 5 minutes then mix the minced onion mixture and set it aside.

Mix the sausage and beef.

Put the meatloaf mixture back into the large mixing bowl and add the egg mixture and mix well. Add the almond mixture and mix well until the meat mixture does not stick.

Cover a cookie sheet with wax paper and place the meat mixture to form a slab shape. Spread the slab with the cream cheese mixture. Fold the meat over the paper and roll it up starting on one end. Cover all the ends to protect the cheese mixture from spilling.

Let this bake until browned at a temperature of 160 degrees F. Leave it for 5-10 minutes and then slice and serve.

20. Asparagus and Chipotle Mayonnaise

Ingredients

2 lbs asparagus

1 chipotle chili, canned in adobo

½ cup mayonnaise

Instructions

Remove the asparagus ends and put them in a microwaveable casserole. Add a few tablespoons of water, and then cover with a plastic wrap. Let this heat for about 6 minutes.

While these are in the oven, place your chipotle and mayonnaise in the food processor. Add a teaspoon of adobo sauce and then turn the food processor on until a smooth sauce is formed.

Serve.

21. Pecans

Ingredients

3 tablespoons butter

2 cups pecan halves

Salt if desired

Instructions

Preheat oven to 350 degrees F. Warm a roasting pan in the oven then melt the butter at the bottom of the warm pan and add the pecans. Stir thoroughly and make sure that the pecans are uniformly coated.

Set the oven timer for 4 minutes and then stir when the four minutes are up. Let them roast for an extra five minutes, and then remove from the oven. Add salt then cool and divide into portions.

22. Curried Pecans

Ingredients

3 tablespoons coconut oil

¼ teaspoon garlic powder

1 teaspoon curry powder

8 ounces pecans

½ teaspoon onion powder

Salt to taste

Instructions

Preheat the oven to 350 degrees F. Put coconut oil in a roasting pan and melt it in the oven while it heats.

Remove the pan from the oven and stir in the seasonings when the coconut oil has melted, and then add the pecans. Blend well by stirring thoroughly until all of them are uniformly coated.

Let these roast for 5 minutes, and then stir and return to the oven for another 4 to 5 minutes. Let them cool, and add salt to taste. Divide into portions and serve.

23. Pork chops

Ingredients

4 pork chops

1 stalk peeled and diced lemongrass

1 medium star anise

1 tablespoon of fish sauce

4 Garlic Cloves

1/2 tablespoon of sugar free ketchup

1 tablespoon of almond flour

1 1/2 teaspoon of soy sauce

1/2 tablespoon of sambal chili paste

1/2 teaspoon mixed spice

1 teaspoon sesame oil

1/2 teaspoon of peppercorns

Instructions

Wrap the pork chops with a rolling pin wrapped in wax paper.

Cut the garlic cloves into halves and place them aside then grind the anise and peppercorns until they form a fine powder using a mortar and pestle. Add garlic and lemongrass and then mix until they form a smooth mixture. Add the soy sauce, fish sauce, mixed spice and sesame oil, and then mix well.

Place pork chops in a tray then coat with the marinade and let these marinate at room temperature while covered for 1-2 hours.

Pre-heat the pan and lightly coat the pork chops in almond flour.

Place them in the pan and turn once when they have seared on one side. They should form a golden brown crust after about 2 minutes under heat.

Cut all the chops into several strips. Make the sauce by stirring in the sugar free ketchup and Sambal chili paste.

Serve with Mashed Potatoes or crisp garlic parmesan green beans.

24. Keto Casserole

Ingredients

1/2 pound corned beef diced

2 cups swiss cheese shredded

1 can sauerkraut drained

1* 8 oz package cream cheese

1/2 cup mayonnaise

1/2 cup low-sugar ketchup

1/2 teaspoon caraway seeds

2 tablespoons pickle brine

Instructions

Preheat oven to 350 degrees F.

Melt the mayonnaise, ketchup and cream cheese, over low heat in a saucepan. Slice the corned beef into big chunks and dice it while the cream cheese is melting.

Add 1 1/2 cups of the swiss cheese, chopped corned beef and the drained sauerkraut when the mixture has melted. Mix until everything has blended completely with the cheese.

Remove the sauce from the heat and blend in the pickle juice if present, or a teaspoon of vinegar, salt and a pinch of garlic salt to taste.

Put this in an oiled dish and add the remaining swiss cheese at the top. You can sprinkle caraway seeds at the top to garnish.

Put in the oven to melt the cheese at the top for about twenty minutes.

25. Baked Salmon

Ingredients

2 cloves of minced garlic

1 teaspoon of dried basil

6 tablespoons of olive oil

1 teaspoon of ground black pepper

1 teaspoon salt

1 tablespoon fresh chopped parsley

1 tablespoon lemon juice

2 salmon fillets

Instructions

Prepare the marinade in a glass bowl by mixing light olive oil, garlic, lemon juice, parsley, salt and pepper. Find a medium sized baking dish to put the salmon fillets and then spread with the marinade. Put this in a refrigerator to marinate for about 1 hour while turning occasionally.

Preheat oven to 375°F; roll the fillets using aluminum foil, spread with marinade and then seal. Put these in a glass dish and slide in an oven until they can produce flakes easily. Serve while hot.

26. Keto Frittata

Ingredients

1 tablespoon of coconut oil

300g of fatty ground beef or any meat of your choice and add bacon

4 eggs

½ red pepper

½ green pepper

4 mushrooms

3 leaves of Kale

1 tablespoon of curry powder

200g of goat cheese

1 tablespoon of garlic powder

1 tablespoon of paprika

Instructions

Cut the mushrooms, kale, red pepper and green pepper into small pieces.

Let the coconut oil melt in a pan under medium heat and sauté the vegetables until set.

Add the ground beef and cook while stirring until it turns brown.

Beat the eggs and blend with the spices.

Spread the ingredients uniformly over the pan before you pour the eggs in the pan.

Add the goat cheese at the top.

Cover the skillet until the cheese starts bubbling and the eggs are cooked. This can take approximately 3 minutes.

27. Fried Chicken

Ingredients

¾ cup of plain whey protein

1 tablespoon of oat fiber

1 cup of crushed pork rinds

½ teaspoon of onion powder

1 teaspoon of salt

1/8 teaspoon of coarse black pepper

½ cup parmesan cheese

¼ cup of heavy cream

2 large eggs

½-3/4 inch deep hot oil

¼ cup of water

Instructions

Mix all the dry ingredients by shaking well in a plastic bag. Mix the cream, water and eggs in a large bowl then add the chopped chicken into the egg wash and coat each piece well by turning several times. Remove each piece from the bowl and coat with the seasoned flour.

Heat ¾ inch deep oil under very high heat. Arrange the pieces next to each other. Coat the other pieces of chicken. Cook until the chicken turns brown on both sides but do not disturb it too much. When brown, remove and let it drain. Cook the rest of the chicken if not all the pieces were able to get in your skillet.

28. Shrimps and Avocadoes

Ingredients

1 cup of shrimps

Half avocado

½ tablespoon of organic peanut butter

Sriracha hot sauce

1 tablespoon of coconut milk

1 teaspoon shredded Coconut

Instructions

Spray the saucepan with an olive oil sprayer on medium temperature then pour the peanut butter, coconut milk, and the Sriracha hot sauce.

Add shrimps and sauté for 4 minutes until the shrimps turn pink.

Slice the avocado into small pieces and put on a plate.

Add the avocados at the top and sprinkle the shredded coconut.

29. Spinach Sardines with tomato soup

Ingredients

2 tablespoons of vegetable or corn oil

1 whole, sliced onion

1 tablespoon, crushed garlic

Spanish sardines in olive oil and tomato sauce

1 large, sliced tomato

1 to 2 cups of fresh spinach

2 to 3 cups of water or vegetable broth

1 teaspoon of black pepper powder

1 teaspoon of salt

Instructions

Pour the vegetable or corn oil in a medium pot with medium high heat.

Sauté the onions, garlic, and tomatoes then let these cook for 3 to 5 minutes until the tomatoes and onions are soft.

Add in sardines and sauté. Break the sardines into small particles to dissolve in the tomato-onion mixture.

Add the broth and let it boil, then lower heat.

Add the salt, pepper and spinach leaves. Cook for 1 to 2 minutes until the spinach turns but is not wilted. Serve hot with jasmine white rice.

Snacks And Side Dishes

30. Deviled Eggs

Ingredients

6 large eggs

¼ teaspoon of french mustard

1 tablespoon of hellman's mayonnaise

A few drops of hot sauce (optional)

1 teaspoon of paprika

1 teaspoon of cumin (optional)

1/2 teaspoon of cayenne pepper (optional)

Salt & pepper to taste

Parsley to garnish

instructions

Remove the yolk from the hardboiled eggs.

Using a fork, mash the yolk and add the other ingredients.

Mix until everything blends in well to form a thick mixture.

Fill the eggs with the mixture and sprinkle paprika at the top.

31. Egg Muffins

Ingredients

6 Eggs

½ cup of Sliced Spinach

6 slices of nitrate free shaved turkey

Mozzarella Cheese

3 tablespoons Red Pepper

2 tablespoons finely chopped red onion

Fresh Basil (optional)

Salt & Pepper

Instructions

Preheat the oven to 350 degrees F.

Slice the red onions, basil, spinach, and red pepper and grate your mozzarella cheese.

Spray a nonstick muffin tin with olive oil spray; gently drop the piece of turkey in one of the cups and let it rest at the bottom and the sides and expand the cup.

Break an egg and pour it into the cup with the turkey.

Add a little of the sliced red onion, spinach, red pepper and cheese on the egg.

Add fresh basil and sprinkle a little pepper and salt onto the egg.

Put the muffin tin in the oven and bake until the eggs are set. If you want the eggs with a runny yolk, then ten minutes should be enough, but a harder one needs at least 15 minutes.

32. Stuffed Mushrooms

Ingredients

1 lb mushrooms

½ cup chicken broth

8 ounces Boursin cheese

Paprika to garnish

Instructions

Preheat the oven to 350 degrees F. Remove the stems from the mushrooms, and reserve them for another use.

Fill all the mushrooms with Boursin, and place them in a baking pan.

Pour some chicken broth around the mushrooms to fill the bottom of the pan. Spread lightly with paprika.

Bake for 30 to 40 minutes and serve hot.

33. Guacamole

Ingredients

1 tablespoon minced red onion

1 ripe avocado

½ garlic clove, crushed

1 tablespoon olive oil

¼ lime

Salt to taste

2 dashes hot sauce, or to taste

½ tablespoon minced cilantro, optional

Instructions

Put the minced onion and crushed garlic in a bowl.

Cut the avocado into two halves and scoop out the flesh using a spoon, then place it (the flesh) in the bowl.

Mush up the avocado using a fork. Don't let it smoothen too much but stop when there are little lumps of the avocado. Squeeze in the lime juice then add the hot sauce, olive oil, salt, and cilantro. Stir and serve immediately.

34. Sweet and Tangy Creamy Pork

Ingredients

2 tablespoons of canned jalapeno pepper slices

1 teaspoon of coconut oil

Liquid sucralose to taste

⅓ ounce pork rinds

¼ cup whipped cream cheese

Instructions

Mix the liquid sucralose with the peppers to get a hot, tangy, and sweet mixture. Set aside while you melt the coconut oil over medium heat, and blend in with the whipped cream cheese.

Be careful not to use too many pork rinds or else you will mess the fat ratio; you can weigh them if you have a scale.

Spread the pork rinds with the cream cheese, add one slice of sweetened jalapeno, and serve.

35. Jalapeno Peppers

Ingredients

2 fresh jalapeno peppers

2 slices bacon

1 ½ ounces cream cheese

Instructions

Prepare the peppers by slitting them and remove the stems and seeds.

Divide the cream cheese into two, and stuff each pepper.

Roll all the peppers in bacon and seal if you can (toothpicks are great to secure it). Make sure to wash your hands thoroughly to remove any pepper left on your hands.

Broil or grill until the bacon is cooked.

36. Fettuccine with Pancetta Cream

Ingredients

1 packet tofu shirataki fettuccini

1 tablespoon butter

1 ounce pancetta (Italian bacon)

1 teaspoon of minced parsley

½ ounce cream cheese

Instructions

Drain and rinse your shirataki, and put them in a bowl. Snip across them using your kitchen shears and then nuke them for two minutes then cut the pancetta fairly fine. Put a medium-sized skillet over medium-low heat, and let the bits to brown.

When the shirataki are done, drain them again, and nuke them for another minute. Stir in the pancetta. After about a minute, drain the noodles again and stir the pancetta.

Add the cream cheese and butter to the noodles, and let them melt to coat the noodles evenly.

Put the crispy pancetta bits and all the fat from the pan into the noodles. Add the parsley, toss once more, and serve.

37. Chocolate Peanut Butter Bombs

Ingredients

3 ounces 85% dark chocolate

3 tablespoons coconut oil

8 tablespoons butter

1 tablespoon heavy whipping cream

4 tablespoons natural creamy peanut butter

½ cup macadamia nuts

Sugar substitute equal to 6 teaspoons of sugar

Instructions

Put the butter and chocolate in the microwave to melt for a few seconds. Add the rest of the ingredients but leave the macadamia nuts and mix until smooth.

Stir in the macadamia nuts and pour about 2 to 3 teaspoons into each paper-baking cup.

Store in freezer.

Eat frozen or warm for 5 minutes.

38. Creamy Strawberry And Pecans

Ingredients

1 tablespoon chopped pecans

French vanilla liquid stevia

⅓ cup sour cream

1 strawberry

Instructions

Stir the chopped pecans in a small, heavy skillet over medium-low heat for a few minutes if necessary; this makes them crispier. Remove from heat.

Sweeten the sour cream with the French vanilla liquid stevia in a small bowl (you can use a little vanilla extract if you don't want it too sweet). Stir until uniformly sweetened.

Slice the strawberry. Top with the strawberry and pecans, and serve.

39. Chicken Noodle Soup

Ingredients

3 tablespoons of coconut oil

4 tablespoons of diced celery

2 tablespoons of chopped onion

2 cups of chicken broth

4 tablespoons of shredded carrot

1 package tofu shirataki

1 teaspoon of chicken bouillon concentrate

Instructions

Melt the coconut oil in a medium saucepan over medium-low heat. Add the vegetables and sauté for about five minutes.

Add the bouillon and chicken broth then mix and bring to a simmer. Reduce the heat, cover, and let it simmer for another 20 minutes until the veggies are soft.

While you wait for these to cook, drain your shirataki noodles and put them in a microwaveable bowl. Nuke on high for 2 minutes, and then drain again. Separate them using kitchen shears for a few seconds.

Add the noodles to the soup when the veggies are soft then let it simmer for another minute and then serve.

40. Asparagus with Wasabi Mayonnaise

Ingredients

½ lb asparagus

¼ teaspoon of wasabi powder

2 tablespoons of mayonnaise

1 pinch of Splenda

¼ teaspoon of coconut aminos or soy sauce

Instructions

Remove the ends of asparagus that want to break naturally then place the asparagus in a microwave steamer. Add a tablespoon of water, cover with a lid or plastic wrap, and put in the microwave on high for 3 to 4 minutes.

Mix the rest of the ingredients together while stirring in a small dish.

When the 4 minutes are up, remove the lid immediately so that the asparagus does not overcook.

You can eat the cooked asparagus right away with the mayo, or you can refrigerate and eat it later.

41. Pumpkin pies

Ingredients

15-ounce of 100% pure pumpkin puree

2 whole beaten eggs

4 ounces of softened cream cheese

½ cup of heavy whipping cream

½ teaspoon of pumpkin pie spice

2 tablespoons of whipped cream

Artificial sweetener that is equal to ¼ cup of sugar

Instructions

Preheat oven to 350 degrees F.

Beat the cream cheese and pumpkin until they form a smooth mixture using an electric mixer. Beat the eggs and add in the heavy cream, pumpkin pie spice, and sweetener.

Grease some ramekins, place them on a cookie sheet, and then pour the mixture. Let this bake for one hour, or until a knife inserted at the middle comes out clean.

Let it cool and then serve, or put in refrigerator until you are ready to eat.

42. Cheddar Garlic Biscuits

The ingredients in this recipe can make up to 37 biscuits. They are low carb and delicious, and you can customize by extending to make a sandwich bun.

Ingredients

2 ½ cups of divided almond flour

5 tablespoons of butter

6 ounces shredded colby jack cheese

2 large eggs

8 oz cream cheese

1 teaspoon baking soda

2 teaspoons granulated garlic

1 teaspoon sea salt

¾ teaspoon xanthum gum

Instructions

Preheat oven to 325F and spread parchment paper on a cookie sheet.

Place 1 cup of the shredded cheese and almond flour in a food processor. Turn it up until everything is finely ground and set aside.

Place the butter and cream cheese in a glass, mixing bowl. Put in the oven until the butter melts slightly before removing and then whisk until it turns glossy and smooth.

Beat in the eggs until the mixture turns smooth and glossy. Blend in the garlic, xanthium gum, baking soda, and salt.

Mix the almond flour-cheese mixture and egg mixture. Add the remaining almond flour and stir until it mixes well and forms dough.

Use a tablespoon to scoop the dough then place it on the cookie sheet, making one-inch gaps. Rolling the dough will smoothen.

Bake for around 25 minutes or until a golden brown color is visible at the top. Remove and leave it for ten minutes to cool.

Bonus Recipes

Cauliflower And Bacon Quiche

Ingredients

2 lb raw cauliflower without the leaves and lower stalk

2 ounces of minced green pepper

4 ounces of minced white onion

4 ounces of cooked and crumbled bacon

1 tablespoon of butter

6 eggs

2 cups of shredded colby jack or cheddar

Salt and pepper to taste

1/2 cup of heavy cream

Instructions

Cut the cauliflower into smaller pieces, including the core. Bring a large pan of water to boil and salt lightly. Turn to medium heat, add the cauliflower and cook until they become completely tender. This should take about 20-30 minutes. You can use a steaming pan combo set to steam the cauliflower.

Use a colander to drain the cauliflower and then set aside.

Melt the butter and sauté the bell pepper and onions over medium heat in a large skillet until they become translucent and soft.

Mince the cauliflower once it has cooled and measure out 3 cups.

Press the excess water from the cauliflower using paper towels, cup, or a sturdy bowl.

Press the cauliflower into a pan, and make sure the crust is uniform and consistent in thickness.

Dip the bacon into the onion-pepper mixture, and spoon-feed it over the cauliflower crust.

Add the shredded cheese at the top of the vegetable layer.

Beat the eggs, and blend them in with the cream and spices until they turn frothy. Pour the mixture over the rest of the ingredients in the pan.

Put in a microwave for 25-35 minutes at 350 degrees, or until the top is golden.

Cauliflower Casserole

Ingredients

2 lb of raw cauliflower without the leaves and lower stalk

1 tablespoon of butter

4 ounces chopped white onion

4 fl oz heavy cream

2 ounces chicken broth

2 cups shredded colby jack or cheddar

4 oz cream cheese

Instructions

Cut the cauliflower into smaller pieces, including the core. Bring a large pan of water to boil and salt lightly. Turn medium heat on, add the cauliflower and cook until they become completely tender. This should take about 20-30 minutes. You can use a steaming pan combo set to steam the cauliflower.

Use a colander to drain the cauliflower and then set aside.

Melt the butter and sauté the bell pepper and onions until they become translucent and soft over medium heat in a large skillet.

Add the cauliflower and break it into smaller pieces with a spoon. Mix in the onion. Turn heat to medium low, and add the heavy cream and chicken broth, while stirring to mix. Blend in the cream cheese until it melts, while adding a little chicken broth where necessary. Add the shredded cheese and stir until it melts and incorporates into the mixture and forms a creamy sauce. Serve or add more cheese then place in the microwave for about 20 minutes to bake.

7-Day Meal Plan

Day One

Breakfast:

Sausage & Spinach Frittata

Coffee with 2 Tbsp of Heavy Cream

Snack

1/2 avocado sprinkled with salt and pepper

Lunch

1/2 cup of simple egg salad

2 slices of cooked bacon

4 lettuce leaves

Snack

24 raw almonds

Dinner

3/4 cup easy cauliflower gratin

6 oz of rotisserie chicken

2 cups of chopped romaine lettuce

2 tbsp of sugar free caesar salad dressing

Dessert

2 Lindt 90% Chocolate

Day Two

Breakfast

Creamed coconut milk with berries and nuts

¼ cup of fresh raspberries, blackberries, or strawberries

½ cup of creamed coconut milk

A handful of almonds

Pinch of cinnamon. Be sure to refrigerate overnight before using it.

Net carbs: 7 g

Lunch

Keto tuna salad

1 tin of tuna (180g)-you can use cooked chicken as an alternative

2 hard-boiled pastured eggs

1 small head lettuce (3.5 oz)

A splash of lemon juice

1 medium spring onion (0.5 oz)

2 tablespoon of home-made mayo (You can make this using healthy oils like macadamia or avocado).

Himalayan salt to taste

Net carbs: 3.9 g

Dinner

One-minute egg muffin- Group everything into 2 cups and put in the microwave for 1-2 minutes

3 large pastured eggs

1 cup frozen spinach (150g / 5.3 oz)

Pink Himalayan salt to taste

Optional: pastured ham, smoked salmon or crispy pastured bacon with two cups of Green salad

2 cups of crispy greens (2.1 oz)

1 avocado (7.1 oz)

1 tbsp of olive oil

Pink Himalayan salt to taste

A splash of lemon juice

Day Three

Breakfast

Omelet prepared using 1 tbsp ghee, 3 large pastured eggs, and pink Himalayan salt complemented with the slow-cooked meat topping (5.3 oz) that you've prepared in advance. Serve with ½ cup of Sauerkraut (2.5 oz).

Net carbs: 3 g

Lunch

Avocado salad

½ avocado (3.5 oz)

2 hard-boiled pastured eggs

1 small head crunchy lettuce (3.5 oz)

A splash of lemon juice

1 medium spring onion (0.5 oz)

1 tbsp of extra virgin olive oil

Pink Himalayan salt to taste

Net carbs: 7.9 g

Dinner

Roasted pork chops with asparagus

1 medium pork chop sprinkled with pink Himalayan salt to season, and pan-roasted using 1 tbsp of ghee or lard (7.1 oz)

1 large bunch of asparagus, seasoned with a splash of fresh lemon juice, salt and pan-roasted using 1 tbsp of ghee (7.1 oz)

Day Four

Breakfast

1 large pastured egg the way you want it, 1 package of pastured ham or smoked wild salmon (3.5 oz), 1 cup of braised spinach (5.3 oz), 1 tbsp of ghee, pink Himalayan salt to taste, 1 cup of fresh or frozen berries (5.3 oz). Of all the berries, blackberries have the least amount of carbs.

Carbs: 8.6 g

Lunch

Quick prawn & spinach salad

1 package of pan roasted prawns with 1 tbsp of ghee (7.1 oz)

¼ cup of green or black olives (1 oz)

2 cups of fresh spinach or other greens such as rocket, lettuce, or chard, (2.1 oz)

Pink Himalayan salt and cayenne pepper to taste

2 tbsp of extra virgin olive oil

Carbs: 2.8 grams

Dinner

Slow-cooked meat with lettuce cups

7.1 oz of slow-cooked meat (200g)

1 cup of cherry tomatoes (5.3 oz)

1 small head crunchy lettuce (3.5 oz)

Tomato salad

1 tbsp of freshly chopped or dried basil

1 medium spring onion (0.5 oz)

Pink Himalayan salt to taste

1 tbsp of extra virgin olive oil

Day Five

Breakfast

2 scrambled eggs (pastured) with 1 small spring onion or a bunch of chives, 3 thick rashers bacon (pastured) or ham (3.2 oz), ½ avocado with pink Himalayan salt (3.5 oz), 1 tbsp of ghee. Serve with ½ a cup of Sauerkraut (2.5 oz).

Total carbs: 4.2 g

Lunch

Quick avocado salad

½ avocado (3.5 oz)

2 hard-boiled pastured eggs

1 small head crunchy lettuce (3.5 oz)

A Splash of lemon juice

1 medium spring onion (0.5 oz)

1 tbsp of extra virgin olive oil

Pink Himalayan salt to taste

Net carbs: 7.9 g

Dinner

Slow-cooked meat with lettuce cups

7.1 oz of slow-cooked meat (200g)

1 small head crunchy lettuce (3.5 oz) with Simple tomato salad

1 cup of cherry tomatoes (5.3 oz)

1 medium spring onion (0.5 oz)

1 tbsp of freshly chopped or dried basil

1 tbsp of extra virgin olive oil

Pink Himalayan salt to taste

Net carbs: 6.7 g

Day Six

Breakfast

2 Cream Cheese Pancakes (8g protein, 14g fat, 1g net carbs, 172 calories)
2 pieces of cooked bacon (6g protein, 0g net carbs, 7g fat, 92 calories)
Coffee with 2 Tbsp of Heavy Cream (0g protein, 1g of carbs, 12g fat, 120 calories)

Snack

2 String Cheese (16g protein, 12g fat, 2g net carbs,160 calories)

Lunch

1/2 cup of "Anti" Pasta Salad (3g protein, 4g net carbs, 8g fat,102 calories)

4 Sundried Tomato & Feta Meatballs (24g protein, 32g fat, 2.5g net carbs,356 calories)

Snack

1 cup of bone broth (1g protein, 1g fat, 0g net carbs, 50 calories)

Dinner

1 cup of Cuban Pot Roast (the taco salad style) (20g protein, 2g net carbs, 19g fat, 271 calories)

2 cups of chopped romaine lettuce (1g protein, 1g net carbs, 0g fat, 16 calories)

2 Tbsp of sour cream (1g protein, 1g net carbs, 5g fat,51 calories)

1 Tbsp chopped cilantro, optional

1/4 cup of shredded cheddar cheese (7g protein, 5g net carbs, 9g fat,114 calories)

Dessert

2 squares Lindt 90% Chocolate (3g protein, 3g net carbs, 9g fat, 105 calories,)

Day Seven

Breakfast

3 eggs (any way you want) (19g protein, 1g net carbs, 14g fat, 215 calories)

1 tsp of butter (0g protein, 0g net carbs, 4g fat, 36 calories,)

2 pieces of cooked bacon (6g protein, 0g net carbs, 7g fat, 92 calories,)

Coffee with 2 Tbsp of Heavy Cream (0g protein, 1g net carbs, 12g fat,120 calories)

Snack

24 raw almonds (6g protein, 2g net carbs, 15g fat, 166 calories)

Lunch

1 cup Cuban of Pot Roast (the taco salad style) (20g protein, 2g net carbs, 19g fat, 271 calories)

2 cups of chopped romaine lettuce (1g protein, 1g net carbs, 0g fat,16 calories)

2 Tbsp of sour cream (1g protein, 1g net carbs, 5g fat, 51 calories) optional 1 Tbsp of chopped cilantro

1/4 cup of shredded cheddar cheese (7g protein, 5g net carbs, 9g fat, 114 calories)

Snack

1 cup of bone broth (1g protein, 0g net carbs, 1g fat, 50 calories)

Dinner

1 1/2 cup of chili spaghetti squash casserole (23g protein, 6g net carbs, 20g fat, 284 calories)

2 cups of raw baby spinach (2g protein, 1g net carbs, 0g fat,14 calories)

1 tablespoon of sugar free ranch dressing (0g protein, 1g net carbs, 7g fat, 70 calories)

Dessert

2 squares Lindt 90% Chocolate (3g protein, 3g net carbs, 9g fat, 105 calories)

Conclusion

The ketogenic diet is fast becoming the easy way to lose weight healthily and quickly. However, this diet was initially meant for people who were struggling with epilepsy, but because of the low carb content in the diet, you can use it to lose weight as well. In addition, there are numerous other health benefits of this diet. One such benefit is that it improves your body's ability to absorb fats and convert them into energy. On the other hand, it reduces the levels of insulin in your body, which in turn causes greater lipolysis and the release of free glycerol unlike the normal diet.

I hope this book will enable you to make healthier choices to enable you achieve your desired weight loss goals.

Thank you again for purchasing this book!

Sara Banks

Disclaimer

Please remember that anything discussed here does not constitute medical advice and cannot substitute for appropriate medical care.

Printed in Great Britain
by Amazon.co.uk, Ltd.,
Marston Gate.